EMOTIONAL FREEDOM TECHNIQUES & TAPPING FOR BEGINNERS

EFT TAPPING SOLUTION MANUAL : 7 EFFECTIVE TAPPING THERAPY TECHNIQUES FOR OVERCOMING ANXIETY AND STRESS

PAUL ROGERS

INTRODUCTION

Our lives are filled with unprecedented levels of stress and anxiety, whether it's our job, family or money worries.

We can feel stressed, angry, struggle to meet deadlines or feel as though we have been badly treated.

These stressors, big or small, can have serious and far-reaching consequences on our lives, whether it's on our health and wellbeing, or our goals and dreams.

Of course, we know that we should deal with the stress, but simply don't have the time or energy.

So, what's the solution to our dilemma?

Emotional Freedom Technique, also known as EFT, is something you can easily learn and integrated into your daily life.

By learning some simple tapping techniques, you'll be able to deal with overwhelm, stress and anxiety in a natural and effective way.

This will allow you to unshackle yourself from depression, anxiety and even some physical pain, and empower you with positive energy and motivation so that you can live the life you've always dreamed of.

If you think this sounds all a bit too crazy to be true, let me say right now, there are several scientific papers have validated the benefits of EFT and tapping techniques.

EFT is holistic therapy that you can do anywhere and at any time by yourself.

It allows you to 'tap' into your body's energy and can reduce or even remove negative emotions which can have a harmful impact on your health.

It combines pressing on meridian (energy) points in the body, with positive affirmations and some of the principles of meditation, which combine together in an effective three pronged attack on underlying health issues.

Peter was highly skeptical about EFT. It all sounded a bit too esoteric. However, circumstances in his life were really bad and he decided to try it, thinking 'Why not?'.

He jumped in with both feet and was committed to trying it for at least 30 days before making any judgments.

To Peter's surprise he found it hugely beneficial and effective. He still practices EFT today.

Research by the Centers for Disease Control and Prevention (CDC) estimates that 85 percent of all disease is caused by negative emotions. That's an astonishing figure!

Our negative emotions release various stress hormones into our bodies, such as cortisol that can negatively affect our immune systems. That's why having a positive attitude is crucial for our health and wellbeing.

EFT works by dealing with the emotional causes that underlie the disease or physical pain.

In today's society too many of us are dependent upon pills to cure illness, whether it's depression or anxiety. This can often present more problems through additional side effects and physical dependency.

One of the great things about EFT is that it is a holistic approach, where no pills are needed. It's something you can try yourself at home, you can start seeing benefits quickly, potentially saving you both time and money.

Despite it's rather scientific start, EFT has been streamlined into an easy yet highly effective self-therapy that anyone can use on their own.

This book includes step-by-step instructions, together with scripts for anxiety and phobias, to help guide you through the routine.

Of course, it's not intended to replace your medical program or advice from your physician, but it can be used in combination with it for greater results.

If you're ready to start your tapping journey to better health and emotional freedom, read on!

ONE
WHAT IS TAPPING?

Let's start by looking at just what tapping is and where the idea originated from.

EFT and Tapping

Emotional freedom therapy (also known as EFT) is a new psychological treatment method, an alternative therapy, which is widely practiced by people all over the world.

Research has shown that EFT is a very effective and efficient method that can help people in multiple ways.

It can help treat psychological issues like stress, anxiety and overcome addictions like smoking, drinking, gambling etc. It can also be helpful in improving self-esteem and self-confidence.

EFT is based on tapping our meridian points and makes use of scripts to overcome and treat problems. You may use this powerful healing technology either by taking support from a therapist or by carrying out the techniques by yourself.

EFT is a type of energy therapy and works in a similar way to other energy therapies, such as acupuncture and acupressure.

It's believed that EFT works by rebalancing energy flow as it moves across channels in your body known as meridians.

Research has shown that EFT taps into a section of the brain that stores and processes data, which is used in neurophysiology.

EFT practitioners believe that negative thoughts linger as blockages in your brain, which could result in an array of symptoms like fear, anger, stress etc.

Some of the causes behind such negative emotions include psychological or emotional disturbances or events.

If you feel that you are inadequately trained, or that the trauma is too intense, or feel there is a lack of progress, then get in touch with a qualified practitioner who can help work on your issues and also offer support and advice on how to improve your own self-practice.

Origins of Tapping

Emotional freedom therapy has its roots based on therapies like Neuro-Linguistic Programming (also known as NLP), Behavioral Kinesiology and Thought Field Therapy (also known as TFT).

There is an interesting story about the origin of Thought Field Therapy, which in turn paved the way for Emotional Freedom Therapy.

Dr. Roger Callahan was a cognitive psychologist and hypnotherapist who specialized in phobias. He was researching about Chinese meridians and their effect when you tap at certain meridian points.

A patient who was suffering from intense phobia of water, came to see Dr. Roger Callahan. He had already tried certain conventional therapies to cure her but was not successful.

She complained that she often feels pain in her stomach even when she just thinks about water and her phobia.

Dr. Roger Callahan asked her to tap beneath her eyes for couple of times (this location corresponds to stomach meridian).

By applying this seemingly simple technique the patient was relieved of the phobia.

Later, Gary Craig who worked with Dr. Roger Callahan in Thought Field Therapy started to apply this technique to his patients.

He improved some techniques and simplified the process and this adapted method became Emotional Freedom Therapy.

TWO
HOW EFT WORKS

The emotional freedom technique uses acupressure and psychology to help improve a person's emotional health.

Even though emotional health tends to be overlooked, it plays a crucial part in a person's physical health and their ability to heal.

It doesn't matter how devoted a person is to maintaining proper lifestyle and diet, if they have emotional barriers standing in their way, they won't achieve the body that they want.

Most of the time, you can apply EFT directly to your physical symptoms to find relief without working through the emotional contributors. However, for a powerful and lasting result, you need to figure out and work through the emotional issues.

The premise of EFT also understands that the more emotional issues you can work through, the more emotional peace and freedom you will have.

With EFT you can get rid of limiting beliefs, increase personal performance, improve relationships, and have better physical health. To be honest, everybody on Earth has a couple of emotional issues that they are holding onto.

EFT is extremely easy to learn and can help you in areas such as:

- achieving positive goals
- eliminating or reduce pain
- reduction of
- food cravings, and
- the removal of negative emotions.

And that's just the beginning of what it can do for you.

EFT is based on the meridians of energy that have been used in traditional acupuncture to heal emotional and physical problems for more than five thousand years, but without using needles.

Instead, it uses simple tapping of the fingertips to move kinetic energy into a specific meridian while you think about your problem and speak an affirmation.

The use of affirmations and tapping the meridians help to clear the emotional block from the bioenergy system. This then helps to restore the body and mind balance that is needed for optimal health.

There are many that are wary of this practice at first, mainly the thoughts of electromagnetic energy that flows through the body.

Then are others that are taken aback by the thoughts of how EFT tapping works.

You need to understand that with this technique you will be tapping with your fingers. There are several acupuncture meridians that live on your fingertips, so when you tap, you are using the energy in your fingertips as well as the energy of the area that you are tapping.

Traditionally the tapping is performed by the index and middle finger and with one hand only. You can use whichever hand that you want.

Many of the tapping points are on either side of your body, so that means you can use whichever side you want, and you can switch sides during a tapping session.

You can also modify the practice by using all of your fingers and both hands to create a gentle, natural curved line. The more fingers you use, them more acupuncture points you will access to.

You will also cover more area so that you can hit the points easier than with a couple of fingers. It's also important that you take off any bracelets or watches that you may be wearing.

Affirmation Statements

Another important part is coming up with the affirmation statement that you will use.

Traditionally, the phrase is something like "Even though I have this (fill in the blank), I deeply and completely accept myself."

You would fill in the blank with a short description of the negative emotion, food craving, addiction, or other problem that you are experiencing.

You can also use the following variations. All of the following are great to use because they use the same basic format. Meaning, they acknowledge what the problem is and create acceptance despite the problem's existence. Those are the things that are important in creating an effective affirmation.

The traditional one is easier to remember, but feel free to use one of the following.

"I accept myself even though I (fill in the blank)," or *"Even though I (fill in the blank), I profoundly and deeply accept myself."*

You can also use *"I accept and love myself even though I (fill in the blank)."*

Some interesting facts about affirmations are:

- you don't have to believe you affirmation truly; all you have to do is say it.

- it's more effective if you can say it with emphasis and feeling, but just saying it will still do the job.
- it's better to speak it out loud, but if you are in public where you need to mutter it or do it silently, it will be just as effective.

You can tune into your problem simply by thinking of what it is.

If you don't tune into your problem, which creates energy disruptions, then EFT will not be effective.

Advice and Caution

You should only ever do what feels right for yours. Never enter into any physical or emotional waters that could be threatening.

It's your job to make sure you stay safe in this setting. You can easily seek professional assistance if you need to.

Here is some advice before you dive into EFT.

1. It is extremely important that you are super specific with your language when you use EFT
2. You have to be completely tuned into your issue. Many times, if you are dealing with something that is very painful, you will try to disconnect from your feelings.
3. Because you are working with energy, it is important to pay attention for a cognitive shift. You will know when one has happened because you will reframe the problem.
4. When you see the problem from a different angle, you will likely be surprised or have a new insight. This is great when this happens, and it may open new, valuable insights.
5. Make sure you stay well hydrated. Water helps to conduct electricity, and you are accessing electrical energy when practicing EFT.

EFT Application Range

The only thing that can limit what EFT can do for you is your imagination.

Experienced practitioners and the EFT originators all over the world, amongst them, are psychotherapists and psychologists, have used EFT on several different issues.

This means that they have used not only with emotional issues, where it works the best, but also for physical issues, with surprising success, whenever there is an emotional component or related traumatic experience.

But that's not the only thing; EFT is also a great tool to use for personal development. It can help to get rid of self-imposed restrictions that prevent people from experiencing abundance, great relationships, wealth, and happiness in their life.

In EFT's short history, it has already been able to help over a thousand people with many common emotional problems, including issues such as:

- confusion, grief, guilt and almost any other emotion you can imagine
- self-doubt
- inner child issues and negative memories
- all types of phobias and fears
- depression
- frustration and anger
- anxiety and stress

The amazing thing is that the benefits don't end there. EFT tapping isn't just limited to getting rid of painful emotions.

It can also help improve your health by:

- increasing feelings of wellbeing
- helping insomnia
- relieving feelings of pain

- reducing physical cravings, for example, for chocolate and cigarettes

It can improve your effectiveness in the things that you do, including:

- give you confidence to speak in front of a crowd and with the people that you are not able to communicate with at the moment
- improve personal and business relationships
- improve your performance in sports, job, and any other areas of your life

Make your quality of life better, including by:

- encouraging spiritual and personal growth
- giving you courage to try things that you have wanted to, but were afraid to
- removing blockages that have kept you from having a life that is full of love and joy

There are many examples of people that have been able to easily recover from emotions that have bothered them for years, and sometimes decades, with the use of EFT.

It has been something that people could turn to for help when nothing else has been able to help them.

It has also successfully helped reduce several physical systems such as insomnia, back pain, and headaches.

The power of EFT is at its best when the physical symptoms are also linked to anxiety and stress.

The developers of EFT had reported a success rate of 80 to 100 percent when it came to emotional problems. When it comes to physical ailments, the percentage of success is somewhat lower.

Most of the time, the effects of EFT are permanent and if they aren't you can easily repeat the process if needed.

It works quickly and is gentle. Often people can release emotions like stress, anger, anxiety, and fear in one session, a few days, or a couple of weeks as compared to months or years when it comes to traditional therapy.

One of the best things about EFT is the fact that it is so versatile. When you master the skills that it takes, which aren't hard, it's almost like developing your superpowers.

You can use these tools in pretty much any situation. Like if you have a big presentation to give at work, or you're going in for a job interview, you can use EFT right before to help calm down your nervousness. It doesn't require anything special, yet it works wonders and can be used anywhere.

THREE
THE SCIENCE & PHILOSOPHY OF EFT TAPPING

EFT tapping is based on the centuries old Meridian System of healing pioneered by the Chinese.

Acupuncture and acupressure, which are forms of Meridian System healing, are now accepted healing techniques validated by acclaimed scientific institutions such as Harvard, Stanford, and other prominent universities and prestigious hospitals in the world.

In a way, since acupuncture and acupressure have already gained acceptance as a healing technique, then we can say so should EFT tapping. After all, EFT tapping is a form of acupressure and acupuncture being based on the Meridian System of healing as well.

If you want more evidence regarding the authenticity and effectiveness of EFT tapping you only need do a bit of research on the internet and you will find a wealth of scientific studies being conducted on EFT tapping.

In a 2012 study into the effects of EFT on stress, subjects were randomly assigned to either an emotional freedom technique (EFT) group, a psychotherapy group receiving a supportive interviews (SI), or a no treatment (NT) group.

The EFT group showed statistically significant improvements in anxiety and depression, compared with the group who received no treatment and were shown to have lower levels of the stress hormone, cortisol.

In another study, to investigate whether Thought Field Therapy (also known as TFT) could have an impact on a variety of anxiety disorders. 45 patients were assigned randomly to either TFT or a control group waiting list.

Those patients assigned to the TFT treatment group showed a significant decrease in all symptoms.

More interesting though was that the significant improvement seen after treatment was still evident on year later, showing that TFT may have an enduring anxiety-reducing effect.

A study in 2013 set out to evaluate the short-term effects of EFT on tension-type headache sufferers. Patients were randomly assigned to one of two groups. Those in the EFT group reported significantly reduced frequency and intensity of headache episodes.

It's early days for the science behind EFT, but of course, it was only a few decades ago that acupuncture and acupressure were considered as weird alternative therapies too.

If you really want to determine how useful EFT tapping is, the best way is to give it a test run and start practicing it.

You, yourself, are the best measure of how effective a healing technique EFT tapping is for your own emotional issues.

The First Discovery Statement, Emotional Healing

The philosophy behind EFT tapping can be summed up in one statement:

The cause of all negative emotions is the disruption in the body's energy system.

Practitioners of EFT tapping disagree with the conventional practice of psychotherapy to relieve traumatic memory again and again in order for the person to heal from their negative emotional effects.

EFT tapping believes it necessary to recognize the memory, in order to heal. However, it is more important to identify how and where in the body the energy system was disrupted by the memory or experience.

Healing should be focused more on identifying the pressure point of the Meridian system that has been disrupted and apply EFT tapping techniques on said pressure point to get the energy flowing as it normally does.

The Second Discovery Statement : Physical Relief

EFT can assist physical healing by resolving underlying energetic or emotional contributors.

EFT practitioners understand that not all physical ailments require tapping into emotional triggers in order for EFT tapping techniques to heal them.

The reason for this is because some physical ailments are merely caused by a disruption to the balance of the energy flow in the system. They are not caused by emotional stress or trauma.

When this happens, healing the physical ailment will only require tapping at the particular pressure point, without focusing the mind on an emotional catalyst.

Some physical illnesses are so basic that all it requires is tapping at the point of the body where the energy circuit is located.

When using EFT tapping to heal the body, mind and spirit it is necessary to distinguish between illness that is caused by emotional stress or a mere physical disruption to the energy flow in the Meridian system of the body.

The reason for this is that EFT tapping healing techniques differ depending on the ailment. Is it caused by emotional trauma or by physical disruption to the energy flow?

To be effective make sure you are able to identify between the two so that you can identify the most effective EFT tapping technique for healing.

EFT Tapping Points : The Energy Meridian

In order to practice EFT tapping and enjoy its health benefits it is first necessary to understand the EFT tapping points or the energy meridian located all around the body.

Below you'll find a list of EFT tapping points, they are the locations of the ends of the energy meridian and are situated just underneath the skin.

These EFT tapping points are very sensitive to the touch. These same pressure points are used by acupressure and acupuncture to bring healing and physical ease to the body.

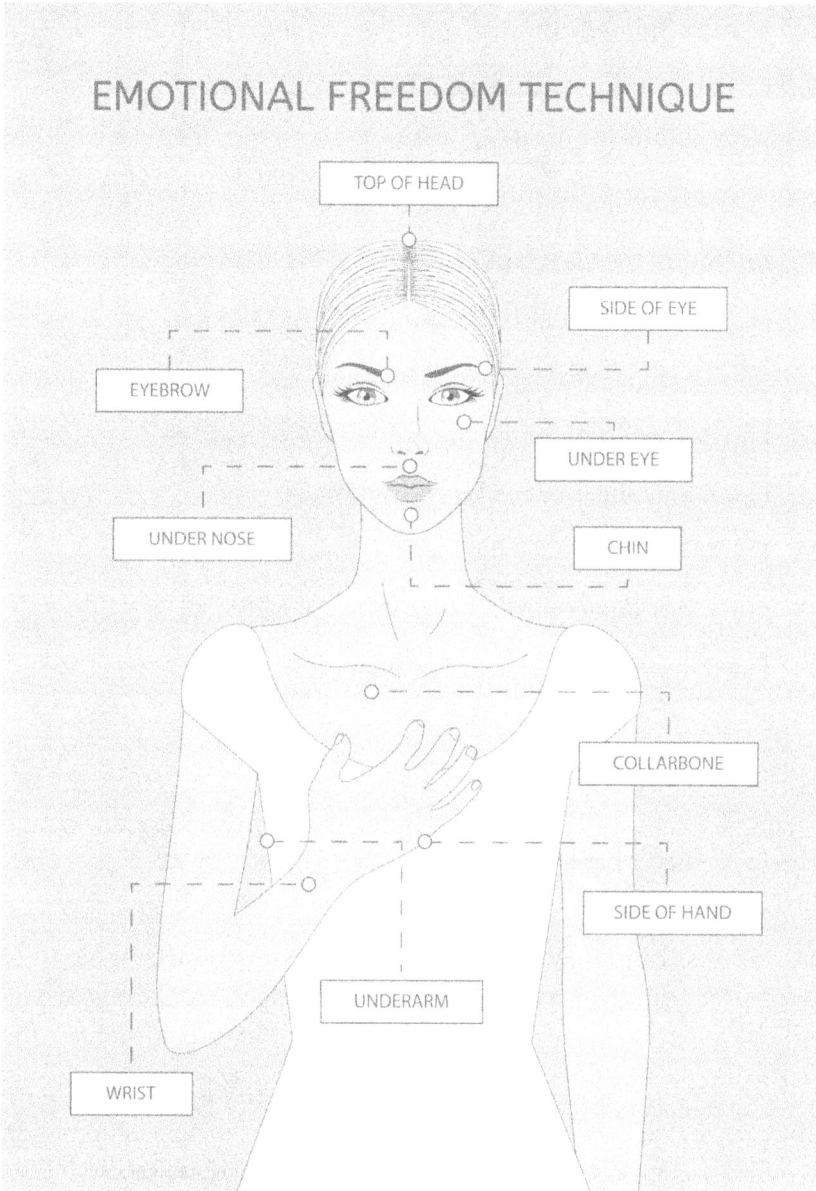

EMOTIONAL FREEDOM TECHNIQUE

Here are the locations of the EFT tapping points:

1. The top of the head or also known as the Governing Vessel

2. The start of the eyebrow or the Bladder Meridian

3. The Sore Spot or the Neurolymphatic Point

4. The side of the eye or the Gall Bladder Meridian

5. Under the eye or the Stomach Meridian

6. Under the nose or the Governing Vessel

7. The chin or the Central Vessel

8. The start of the collar bone or the Kidney Meridian

9. Below the nipple or the Liver Meridian

10. The Karate Chop or the Small Intestine Meridian

11. The Baby Finger or the Heart Meridian

12. The Middle Finger or the Heart Protector

13. The Index Finger or the Large Intestine Meridian

14. The Thumb or the Lung Meridian

15. Under the arm or the Spleen Meridian

Each of these tapping points is connected to a specific and key organ of the body. This means that the body's organs are the energy circuit points where energy flows to, in order to keep the body healthy.

It would be helpful for you to learn and memorize which organ of the body every EFT tapping point is connected to. This way, you will be able to zero in on the EFT point in order to heal the particular part of the body that is ailing.

For example, if you have a migraine, it could be beneficial to tap on the EFT points located in the head area for immediate relief.

If you are looking for complete and long term healing, it is best to cover all 15 EFT tapping points in one session. The same way a full body massage, or full body acupressure session, brings over all relief to the entire body, mind and soul, a full body EFT tapping session can have the same comprehensive easing of tension and stress throughout the body.

Some people find the below-the-nipple EFT tapping point a bit of an awkward tapping point to cover. It is alright to skip this part during your EFT tapping session. But it may come in handy when you have health issues to address that affect the Liver Meridian. When you do it is necessary to tap the below the nipple EFT tapping point.

A special EFT tapping point that is not included in the list is called the Gamut. It is located in the back of both hands and is behind & between the knuckles just at the base of the ring finger. It is an important EFT tapping point that is connected to the heart, the lungs and the liver.

Go ahead stand in front of the mirror and locate all 16 EFT tapping points.

It is necessary to familiarize yourself first about where each tapping point is located. It is a good and necessary start to practicing EFT tapping techniques.

How do I tap?

Let's look at how you actually start tapping.

When you're tapping on the karate cap point, that is, the side of your hand (on the opposite side to your thumb), use all four fingers of your other hand.

When you're tapping on your face, just use your index and middle finger together, to tap gently against your skin.

When tapping your collar bone, you can use the palm of your hand.

Remember, you're going to be tapping on the bony areas. To give you an idea, here's a typical routine you might follow for one round of tapping:

Eyebrow - tap from the inner edge of the eyebrow, above the bridge of you nose, then move across to the *Side of the eye* (between the outer edge of your eye and your hairline) - tap here, moving around until you're tapping *underneath the eye* (below the pupil of your eye, just on the edge of your cheekbone) - tapping gently with two fingers *underneath the nose* (between the bottom of your nose and the upper lip) - tapping gently on the *chin* (on the crease between your lip and chin) using two fingers.

Then move to the *collar bone*, using the palm of your hand to tap *under the arm* (about a hands width below your armpit), tap using four fingers or the palm of your hand.

Finish by tapping the *top of the head*, using just two fingers.

That's what you're going to do, for each round of tapping, as you say the words, which we'll look at later on.

Typically, you'll go through several rounds of tapping, as you:

- *Express* the problem
- *Understand* the problem
- *Explore* the possibilities and what you could change or do
- *Relax* - start using positive, calming words
- *Slow down* - express how you can slow down
- *Choose calm and peace* - affirm the positive

In chapter 5, you'll find some tapping scripts which are helpful for beginners to start with. These scripts are designed so you can just follow the words and tap along.

After you've done this a few times, you'll build up the confidence to start using your own words and express your own feelings, as you tap through the familiar points on your body.

FOUR

HOW DOES TAPPING COMPARE TO OTHER THERAPIES?

Before we get into the detail of using EFT, let's take a quick look at some of the other therapies that relate to the emotions, health and wellbeing.

Neuro-Linguistic Programming (NLP)

Neuro-linguistic programming (also known as NLP) was developed by Richard Bandler and Dr. John Grinder in the 1970s, and is used by people all over the word for resolving both personal and business issues.

NLP is comprised of numerous techniques that affect the way you communicate with yourself and how you could potentially influence communication in others.

This therapy also teaches you how one person's negative thoughts affect them and how these thoughts could be transformed into positive ones.

As the name implies, there is a connection between the neurological process, language and behavioral patterns, which is used to bring about positive changes in life. Like EFT, this treatment is also helpful in treating problems like phobias, depression, anxiety etc.

It involves a lot of visualization if you're interested in motivation and requires you to visualize with as many of your senses as possible.

If you're having issues with anxiety then there are techniques that teach about models and how each person has a different concept of reality. There's also reframing which is a useful technique in change perspectives on certain events.

Theta Healing

This method of treatment was created by Vianna Stibal in 1995 as a way to heal herself from a critical ailment. Theta healing is based on magnetic forces and its connection with your subconscious mind.

For instance, when someone encourages you by saying, "You have done a good job", how does it make you feel?

You would most likely feel energized and motivated. This positive self-talk is one of many techniques used in theta healing.

Theta healing revolves around four key points – core beliefs, genetic, history and soul. Briefly, these are:

- *core beliefs* - these are the beliefs that dwell in your subconscious mind from birth to the present
- *genetic* - this is based upon traits you have inherited from your parents and ancestors
- *history* - this includes assurances, promises, and memories from your present or past life
- *soul*- which refers to the real you, the one that stays even after you die

Electrical signals are produced in your brain, which is measured in the unit hertz. If you enter into theta brainwave, theta healing can occur.

Theta healing can help you to overcome emotional blocks, get rid of genetic and family patterns of beliefs and can help to heal physical ailments.

- *Beta waves* (14–20 hertz): This is regarded as the normal waking conscious level where you are performing routine activities.
- *Alpha waves* (8–13 hertz): This is regarded as a state of light meditation and it is similar to daydreaming.
- *Theta waves* (4–7 hertz): This is regarded as a state of creativity or is similar to a deep meditative state. This is the level that you would be when you are performing theta healing.
- *Delta waves* (1.5–3 hertz): In this wave level, you would be in a deep sleep, unconscious, or in a deep state of meditation.

FIVE

TAPPING FOR OUR EMOTIONS

EFT is a powerful tool that can help you understand more about yourself, your strengths, your weakness. It can help you overcome emotional issues and improve relationships.

Before we get started, let me remind you that this book is not intended as a substitute for the medical advice of physicians.

The reader or listener should regularly consult a physician in matters relating to his/her health and particularly with respect to any symptoms that may require diagnosis or medical attention.

In this chapter we'll go into more details and depth on specific issues, including relationships, stress, fears and anxieties, phobias and depression.

Relationship Issues

One of the basic needs of every human being is to be loved.

When someone feels that he or she is neglected and feels unloved, it naturally creates relationship issues, depression and low self esteem.

We have a natural tendency to be attracted to others who have similar personality traits.

For example, if you value honesty you are more likely to attract and be attracted to an honest person. If you love yourself you would then you are more likely to meet and attract others towards you.

However, if you hate yourself then you are creating barriers that prevent others from getting close to you and entering your life. Negative feelings like jealousy can seriously harm personal relationships and needs to be addressed.

If you feel that, you are jealous or harbor any negative thoughts either towards yourself or your partner then it's most likely than these thoughts or feelings are also having a negative impact on your relationship.

The first step to addressing these issues is to take ownership of them.

Whether you have issues getting close to someone, want to leave a relationship, cope with jealousy, anger or another negative emotion then you can follow the steps below.

Tapping Script for Relationship Issues

Below are examples of setup scripts you can use for the tapping procedure. Feel free to modify them so they fit and reflect your own needs.

Even though I am afraid of getting close, I accept my flaws and myself and would be able to overcome these issues.

Even though I had abusive relationships in past, I accept that I can be a better partner and could master courage.

Even though I get jealous, I love and accept myself completely.

Next, tap on your energy meridian points, starting with the karate chop point and then moving down from the head, while reciting your phrase.

Repeat the process and check how well you feel. Do you feel less jealous? Are you more comfortable in the relationship? If you need to, you can repeat the process again.

How to Deal with Personal Differences in a Relationship

When you are in a relationship, there is often a great of personal issues that arise that you will need to take care of, for both you and your partner.

Spending quality time together and speaking openly about personal differences can help you overcome certain obstacles in the relationship.

Tapping to Deal with Personal Differences in a Relationship

Both of you need to sit down together and list down the good qualities you like in your partner.

Next, write down the qualities you do not like in your partner. I'm aware that this will be difficult, but it's best to be honest.

Then, write down what all experiences in your relationship made you feel happier (like surprise gifts).

Now, talk with your partner about what you wrote down, emphasizing your good qualities and being honest about the bad.

Formulate setup phrases like *"Even though I feel lonely when he is at work, I know that he loves me"* or *"Even though we argue, I know that she loves me"*.

It is a good practice to start with a more insignificant issue.

You may end the process by tapping together. You can also use tapping scripts like *"We love each other and we will work together on our flaws"*.

Stress

Stress is considered the slow and silent killer. It's effects on the body not only reduce your mood but can compromise your immune system.

Science has shown that stress can reduce life expectancy and it's becoming a bigger problem, affecting more and more people every day.

Today, one of the main causes of stress is work, which can lead to anxiety and depression, in addition to stress.

By effectively utilizing EFT in your day-to-day life, you can fight back at stress.

Here's a few benefits of using EFT and tapping to cope with stress:

- you can feel more motivated and more easily able to achieve your targets
- you can be better able to cope with your anger issues
- you can become more capable of adapting to different situations
- you can be able to work better with your colleagues and clients

Now, let's look at a practical way to put this into action.

Tapping Routine for Stress

Say these phrases while tapping the karate chop point of your hand:

Even though I feel overwhelmed by the number of things I have to do, I will find peace and clarity.

Even though problems will be created if I don't finish this soon, this unnecessary stress is making me feel overwhelmed, and I want to find peace and quiet.

Even though I have many things to do, I can be more mindful from now on, about what I commit to and what I delegate.

Tap the points of your body whilst saying out loud the sentences on the right.

Round 1: Express the Overwhelm

Top of the head

I have so many things to do!

Eyebrow

I feel so overwhelmed!

Side of the eye

How am I supposed to get everything done?

Under the eye

I can't believe how much I need to do

Under the nose

It feels as though I have to climb a massive mountain

Chin

It seems as though I will never be able to climb to the top

Collar bone

There's so much to do I don't even know where to start

Under the arm

I will be able to start once I have some clarity

EFT Round 2: Understanding the Overwhelm

Top of the head

I can think much more clearly when I'm not feeling pressured

Eyebrow

My head feels it's spinning from the amount of tasks I need to do

Side of the eye

This is not life or death. Where is the urgency coming from?

Under the eye

Not all of these tasks are urgent

Under the nose

Some of them need to be done now

Chin

Some of them can be done later

Collar bone

Only a few of them are urgent

Under the arm

Worrying about everything at the same time is nonsense

EFT Round 3: Exploring the Possibilities

Top of the head

I'm only creating more pressure on myself

Eyebrow

Wouldn't it be great if everything fell into place?

Side of the eye

Like the pieces of a puzzle?

Under the eye

Without me having to stress out

Under the nose

Maybe I can prioritize the tasks

Chin

So the most important ones get done

Collar bone

I will be able to care of those

Under the arm

And feel great for having accomplished something important

EFT Round 4: Relaxing

Top of the head

If I just focus on the things of importance

Eyebrow

Then I can reduce the feeling of overwhelm

Side of the eye

Because this feeling is negatively affecting me

Under the eye

And reducing my ability to work

Under the nose

Which is only taking me further away from my goal

Chin

I'm smart enough to prioritize things

Collar bone

I'm going to slow down and focus

Under the arm

And create an effective to do list

EFT Round 5: Slowing Down

Top of the head

I just have to slow things down

Eyebrow

There's no to rush through everything

Side of the eye

Things will get done when I'm calm and have clarity

Under the eye

There is great power on being clear about

Under the nose

Knowing what needs to be done

Chin

I'm going to slow down now and focus

Collar bone

This stress is not helping me

Under the arm

I have more control when I'm calm and relaxed

EFT Round 6: Choosing Peace and Calm

Top of the head

I choose to release this stressful energy

Eyebrow

And to focus on doing things that I can do now

Side of the eye

I'm letting go of this feeling of overwhelm

Under the eye

I choose to have a clear mind

Under the nose

I'm going to feel more relaxed and focused

Chin

With every breath I take in and out

Collar bone

I choose to feel good knowing that I'm smart and responsible

Under the arm

I choose to feel calm, confident and powerful

As before, feel free to adapt the wording to suit your own personal circumstances.

Fear and Anxieties

A certain level of fear and anxiety can be healthy. Fear can safeguard you from dangers while healthy levels of anxiety can help you be organized and ready for anything bad that may happen.

However, when fear is unfounded or irrational and it affects your day-to-day life, then it needs to be remedied. It could potentially undermine your physical and emotional health.

Today, there are a lot of people around the world who suffer from different types of phobias like fear of spiders, fear of war, fear of socializing, fear of heights etc.

Phobia is an excessive or irrational fear of certain objects or situations. People suffering from a phobia usually go out of their way to avoid the stimulus that triggers their fear.

How to Handle Fear and Anxiety with the help of EFT and Tapping

If you are suffering from fear, phobias or anxiety and if the traditional techniques haven't worked for you, then you should definitely try EFT which has helped me people overcome this disorders.

Tapping to Deal with Fear and Anxiety

Rate your anxiety/fear level on a scale of 1 to 10 (A rate of 10 denotes that issue is most difficult to cope with).

Identify at what point of time you started to develop this fear. If you are not able to think of the root cause, or when you actually started to develop this fear, you may simply ignore this step.

In the latter case, you may frame the tapping script like "*Even though I don't know the cause for the fear, I still accept and love myself*".

Try to visualize the situation that triggers the anxiety/fear in your mind.

Use an EFT tapping script based on your situation to help you overcome the fear or anxiety.

"Even though I have this anxiety a lot of the time, I accept how I feel and still love myself."

Remember you should be tapping your karate chop point whilst you recite this.

Then tap through the other points on your body starting with the top of the head and working your way down and use a reminder phrase like *"I have this anxiety"*.

Rate your anxiety level again (on a scale of 1 to 10, where a rate of 10 denotes that issue is most difficult to cope with).

Evaluate how your anxiety level is compared to before practicing tapping.

You may need to repeat the tapping process couple of times depending on the intensity of the issue.

Anxiety Script

After you have finished tapping and reciting your setup phrase like *"Even though I have this anxiety a lot of the time, I accept how I feel and still love myself"* you can use the following script for tapping instead of using the reminder phrase.

For it to be most effective, replace the sentences with your own thoughts and feelings.

Here's a script to start putting the theory into action.

EFT Round 1: Express the Anxiety

Top of the head

These anxious feelings that I have

Eyebrow

Are difficult to live with

Side of the eye

There is something I need to do

Under the eye

But this anxiety leaves me feeling paralyzed

Under the nose

It's standing in the way of my success

Chin

It cripples me and leaves me scared

Collar bone

To try new things, go to new places

Under the arm

Or meet new people

EFT Round 2: Understand the Anxiety

Top of the head

I know these feelings

Eyebrow

Are supposed to protect me and prepare me

Side of the eye

But they are just limiting me

Under the eye

They are leaving me afraid

Under the nose

I find it difficult to let go

Chin

The more I think about my anxiety the more it grows

Collar bone

Is something wrong with me?

Under the arm

What can I change?

EFT Round 3: Explore the Possibilities

Top of the head

Focusing on the anxiety is making it worse

Eyebrow

I keep focusing on what will go wrong

Side of the eye

These thoughts are in my head

Under the eye

And they start with me

Under the nose

If I can shift my focus

Chin

And my attention

Collar bone

To something more positive

Under the arm

I can create more positive thoughts

EFT Round 4: Relaxing

Top of the head

I just need to breathe

Eyebrow

And regain my composure

Side of the eye

These thoughts are in my head

Under the eye

Start with me

Under the nose

I will focus on feeling calm

Chin

And relaxed

Collar bone

The slower I breathe in and out

Under the arm

The more relaxed I become

EFT Round 5: Slowing Down

Top of the head

I just have to slow things down

Eyebrow

When I am calm and clear

Side of the eye

I will be able to perform better

Under the eye

Because my worries and angst

Under the nose

Will disappear

Chin

I'm going to slow down now and relax

Collar bone

This anxiety is not helping me

Under the arm

I'm much more in control when I'm calm and relaxed

EFT Round 6: Choosing Calm and Clarity

Top of the head

I choose to release this anxious energy

Eyebrow

And to focus on a positive outcome

Side of the eye

When I let go of these fears and doubts

Under the eye

I will be able to succeed to a greater degree

Under the nose

When I'm relaxed and focused

Chin

I can do and achieve anything

Collar bone

I choose to feel good knowing that I'm smart and responsible

Under the arm

I choose to feel calm, confident and powerful

OK, let's move on to a script to help deal with specific phobias.

Phobia Script

After you have finished tapping and reciting your setup phrase like *"Even though I have this fear of needles, I accept how I feel and still love myself"* you can use the following script for tapping instead of using the reminder phrase.

Of course, for it to be more effective you should replace the sentences with your own thoughts and feelings.

EFT Round 1: Express the Phobia

Top of the head

This phobia that I have

Eyebrow

Is difficult to live with

Side of the eye

It makes me feel embarrassed

Under the eye

It's difficult to talk to people about

Under the nose

It makes going to the doctors a fearful experience

Chin

I worry I will faint

Collar bone

And make a scene

Under the arm

And embarrass myself further

EFT Round 2: Understand the Phobia

Top of the head

I know this feeling

Eyebrow

Is supposed to protect me and prepare me

Side of the eye

But it's just limiting me

Under the eye

It's leaving me afraid

Under the nose

To receive important medical treatment

Chin

Or donate blood for a good cause

Collar bone

No one else I know has this issue

Under the arm

What can I change?

EFT Round 3: Explore the Possibilities

Top of the head

Focusing on the negative outcome

Eyebrow

Is just adding power to my fear

Side of the eye

Every time I put off a check up

Under the eye

Because of the fear

Under the nose

I also reinforce that fear even more

Chin

If I can change my focus

Collar bone

To a more positive outcome

Under the arm

Then I can create more positive thoughts and reduce the fear

EFT Round 4: Relaxing

Top of the head

I just need to breathe

Eyebrow

And regain my composure

Side of the eye

These thoughts that are in my head

Under the eye

Start with me

Under the nose

There is nothing to fear

Chin

Nothing bad is going to happen

Collar bone

I just need to breathe in and out

Under the arm

And allow my mind to become more relaxed

EFT Round 5: Slowing Down

Top of the head

I just have to slow things down

Eyebrow

When I am calm and relaxed

Side of the eye

I can focus more on a positive outcome

Under the eye

Which will allow my worries

Under the nose

To disappear

Chin

I'm going to slow down now and relax

Collar bone

This fear is not helping me

Under the arm

It's standing in my way

EFT Round 6: Choosing Calm and Confidence

Top of the head

I choose to release this fearful energy

Eyebrow

And to focus on a positive outcome

Side of the eye

When I let go of these fears and doubts

Under the eye

I will become more confident

Under the nose

When I'm relaxed and confident

Chin

I can do and achieve anything

Collar bone

I choose to feel good knowing that I'm brave and courageous

Under the arm

I choose to feel calm, confident and powerful

Before reading further, please remember that this book is not intended as a substitute for the medical advice of physicians.

Finally, let's look at how EFT might help with depression.

Depression or Depressive Thoughts

Today, depression is affecting more and more people, especially in the western world. It can cause us to feel empty, sad and hopeless, which in turn drastically reduces our happiness in life.

Depression is thought to block positive energy and depletes our willpower living us unmotivated to carry out even the simplest of daily activities.

However, using EFT and tapping may help combat depression.

A good example of an EFT setup script that you may use if you suffer from depression would be *"Even though I currently suffer from depression, I accept that I will be able to overcome this situation and do well in my life"*.

DEPRESSION SCRIPT

After you have finished tapping and reciting your setup phrase like *"Even though I feel depressed, I accept how I feel and still love myself"* you can use the following script for tapping instead of using the reminder phrase.

As always, feel free to replace the sentences with your own thoughts and feelings, to make it more personal and effective.

EFT Round 1: Express the Depression

Top of the head

This sadness that I have

Eyebrow

Is difficult to live with

Side of the eye

It makes me feel hopeless

Under the eye

It really wears me down

Under the nose

It makes everything seem colourless

Chin

It's sapping my energy

Collar bone

And draining my happiness

Under the arm

It's difficult to open up about it

EFT Round 2: Understand the Depression

Top of the head

What is causing this feeling?

Eyebrow

What is the source?

Side of the eye

Why is it affecting me?

Under the eye

This depression

Under the nose

Is robbing me of my happiness

Chin

And positivity

Collar bone

It's not serving me

Under the arm

How can I fix it?

EFT Round 3: Explore the Possibilities

Top of the head

I need to see the good in life

Eyebrow

And open myself up to good opportunities

Side of the eye

With both my mind and my heart

Under the eye

Even if things feel difficult to do

Under the nose

They will get easier with time

Chin

If I can change my focus and attitude

Collar bone

To a more positive outcome

Under the arm

Then I can live life more fully

EFT Round 4: Opening Up

Top of the head

I'm willing

Eyebrow

To listen and try new things

Side of the eye

I'm willing

Under the eye

To move on with my life

Under the nose

And leave this sadness behind me

Chin

It serves no purpose

Collar bone

It only drains me

Under the arm

My future can be bright again

EFT Round 5: Choosing Confidence and Hopefulness

Top of the head

I choose to release this negative energy

Eyebrow

And to focus on a positive outcome

Side of the eye

When I let go of this sadness and negativity

Under the eye

I will become more confident and hopeful

Under the nose

When I'm confident and hopeful

Chin

I will become re-energized with life again

Collar bone

Positivity and energy will replace my depression

Under the arm

I will live a good and happy life

Next Steps

OK, so you've read through the scripts and you've probably identified which one you feel is probably the best for you.

In order to experience change and start to see benefits, you need to make a decision.

That is, to start actually tapping.

At first, it may seem strange. But, with persistence, you can start feeling calmer and more in control of your emotions.

To really feel the benefit, you'll want to set aside to tap regularly.

By making tapping a habit, it becomes more than a Band-Aid or plaster to use when your emotions get the better or you, or spill over.

If you haven't started yet, when can you set aside 5-10 minutes for your first tapping session?

Once you start to feel the benefits, can you set aside a little time each day to go through the script you feel is most appropriate for that day?

Why not get started today?

SIX
7 WAYS TO USE TAPPING TODAY

In our busy, modern day to day lives there are emotional issues common to everybody. With the pressure of personal finance,

keeping up with friends and family and being constantly on the go, it's easy to see how people can feel lost and discouraged in modern life.

EFT can give you the power to tap away emotional issues affecting day-to-day mindset and performance.

Let's be honest for a moment. How many times have you felt a little out of control over the last week? More often than we'd like to say probably.

We all feel the pressure of busy modern life, but if we let our emotions get control of us, situations can quickly get out of control.

Start by using EFT in your day-to-day routine, whenever the emotions start to take over. With tapping, you can help yourself feel safer, more confident and more self aware so you can continue getting on with your day.

Here are seven of the most common day-to-day applications of tapping.

1. Anger

Anger, frustration, stress, annoyance and all the associated emotions can make up big parts of modern busy life.

Perhaps for you it is a difficult relative, child, boss or co-worker or even road rage that starts you off feeling angry.

Feeling like your space has been breached or offended will bring up negative, angry feelings that can totally change your mood and day.

Here's an example of how EFT changed Andy's life:

Before Andy used EFT, the smallest of slights would set him off. Andy had a closed, self preserving view of the world where everyone could be out to get him at any time!

So whenever someone pushed in line, overtook him on the freeway or spoke bluntly, he was angry that he wasn't being treated fairly. After this anger, it would take hours before he could return to a normal state of mind.

With EFT, Andy was able to tone down his frustrations and cool his anger so he could continue with the day. Before he knew it, what had made Andy angry would slide away like water off a duck's back.

He discovered that there is no better retaliation to anger than overcoming it and getting on with your day!

Learning to overcome anger is something you can do with EFT.

When tapping your sequence, it helps to acknowledge and explicitly state what set you off.

Try this and some of these other phrases to rein in feelings of frustration:

- I am angry at my {spouse, child, co-worker, etc.}
- I am frustrated and angry
- This anger will stop me from doing what I need to do

- I can't afford this anger
- This anger, I can let it go

2. Impatience

With the boom in our economies and globalization, it's not a far stretch to have to wait everywhere we want service.

There's queues at the checkout, queues on the phones, queues to get into restrooms, restaurants, queues in traffic – there's simply no escaping waiting.

Impatience is that itching feeling when you need something right away. And oh, boy does it suck when you're engulfed with nothing but impatience.

Here's an example of how EFT changed Sue's life, in her own words:

"I can attest one area of my life I really struggled with impatience was with online shopping.

I'd spend hours and days browsing the online stores, comparing models, and considering exchange rates and shipping prices to find the perfect purchase.

Only after I paid did I realize it would take more than a week to get the item in my hot little hands. More than a week… outrageous!

If the parcel came when I wasn't home, that'd be another day to pick it up from the post office. In the week the parcel would be in transit I'd wait impatiently, fidgety and not in a good mood.

Impatience was controlling me!"

If you find impatience featuring in your life, here's some EFT tapping phrases you can use.

- I feel impatient, but that's okay
- I really want (whatever I want) now, but I can wait
- I still have a day to get on with
- I won't let impatience stop me from my day

- My life will go on while I wait

3. Worry

With the convenience of modern life, we all feel as if we're under way more pressure.

All this pressure leads to a very stressful, 21st century life! Things weren't as fast paced as they were a couple of decades ago.

We now need to worry about the looming spectre of redundancy, our ability to pay bills and the physical and financial security of ourselves and our loved ones.

When worry plagues the mind, action takes a back seat. Worry hijacks our emotional centres, it rocks the core foundation of our being.

How can you take risks when all you are worried about is the negative outcomes? How can you enjoy life when all that's there is danger? These are the pitfalls of a worrisome life.

Here's what Harry said about his own experience of living with worry:

I know how much worry can control your life. I used to always worry about my financial situation. Several years ago I moved for work, far from family and friends.

Soon after, the company I worked for went through tough times, leaving me worried every day for my job, my livelihood, my rent and my bills.

Worry stopped me from exploring alternate routes to making money.

Only after EFT tapping could Harry overcome his worries, break free from the salary and become the writer and lifestyle coach he is today!

With the emotional freedom technique, you can minimize your worries away to start taking those risks that will help you achieve emotional freedom.

Here's some EFT tapping phrases you can use:

- I am worried about my situation
- I know what I want, but worry is stopping me
- I can overcome my worries
- I will not let worry stop me from taking action
- I am confident and feel secure in myself

4. Low Self-Esteem

Low self-esteem is one of the biggest issues people face every day.

Modern life dangles the image of perfection in front of us with

every sitcom, movie, reality show, advertisement and magazine.

Physically, magazines demand we have the "perfect abs" or the "firm butt" to get the man or woman we want.

Advertisements sell us lifestyles that we can only dream of, being the envy of family and friends with a big new home, driving along rolling hills in our brand new SUVs, being successful with a new watch or fragrance … the list goes on!

The main message these images sell to you and I, is that we are not good enough as we are right now.

Unfortunately, the adverts won't be going away any time soon, but there is one way we can preserve our self-esteem when that nagging feeling emerges. Yes, you've guessed it, EFT tapping!

Low self esteem can come from nasty self perceptions within us too. These self perceptions are often borrowed from childhood or some other twisted source. And the truth is, they simply aren't true.

It is shown again and again that we can be most hard on themselves when it comes to self esteem.

However, as a free thinking and self directing adult, you now can start to address your false perceptions of self through EFT.

Try using these phrases whenever low self esteem tries to creep into your life:

- *I don't feel confident in my own skin*
- *I feel like I need to change, but I am perfect as I am now*
- *I am content with my life and myself*
- *I decide what I need in my life*
- *I have the self esteem I need*

5. Restlessness

Restlessness and lack of sleep is a huge problem in our modern society.

Work has started to follow people home with the mainstreaming of the internet and smart phones. Fizzy energy drinks, caffeine pills, tea, coffee, alarm clocks, fatigue and being on the edge are all symptoms that we, as a culture, have given away precious sleep in exchange for busyness.

So what happens when our head hits the pillow at the end of a busy day?

Well, if you're anything like me back in the day, you'd toss and turn, feel fidgety, be aware of every second that went by and think of what still needed to be done.

Modern life makes it difficult to get to sleep! But with the emotional freedom technique, you may find it easier rest at night.

EFT can help you calm down the nervous system and quiet your mind to get proper rest.

When you tap away your restlessness, try these additional techniques:

Breathe deeply and consciously

Squeeze your eyelids shut and with your eyeballs, direct them up and inside to the middle of your brow. This activates alpha waves in your brain for deep relaxation.

When you open your eyes, focus them on a point in the distance, either out the window or on your roof.

After these additional techniques you can use EFT to tap away your restlessness. Try these mantras or variations for them to get to sleep quickly!

- I am feeling restless
- But my body and mind feels active
- This restlessness means I will not get sleep
- I need relaxing and restful sleep
- I give myself permission to sleep

6. Fear of Success or Failure

Fear of success and fear of failure are the biggest negative blocks to achieving the life we desire.

Here's something of Paul's story:

For years I was terrified of leaving my job to start my own business. I was too scared of the implications of failing in my business idea.

I'd often ask "What would it mean about me, if my own business failed?" and "What would others think if I failed?"

And on the flip side, the fear of success kept me in a day job: "What would I do with all that money?", "Success isn't for me. After all I only come from a working, middle class background"

Fear gripped me into a state of stasis where I was happy just receiving a consistent monthly pay cheque.

Only when I learnt the controlling grip of fear of failure and success could I step away from my passive, "go with the flow" attitude and direct my life.

If you have a fear of failure or success, you must evaluate your beliefs about failing, money and business.

Look back into your childhood and past to see where these beliefs were formed. If there are any negative emotions there, those are the ones you can target!

Blast those negative feelings away with some EFT phrases:

- I am afraid of failure/success
- I feel I don't deserve success/failure is not acceptable
- Failure is not defeat/Success is not evil

7. Procrastination

Perhaps the most negative use of time in our modern lives is when procrastination takes over.

I bet you've been there too, 10 minutes of television ends up being 30 minutes and before you know it, your whole night's gone!

Or you wake up in the morning and waste half an hour or an hour just checking your social media, before you even get out of bed.

Technology takes centre stage in our lives. And although technology has increased our productivity and efficiency, our easy access to the internet has made procrastination that much easier, making us less productive!

If we're not careful, a little 'break' at our computers to read the news, watch a movie or check social media ends up wasting a whole hour or maybe far more!

What's worse is when we procrastinate, the time spent often isn't even very enjoyable.

Time spent procrastinating is different to time spent in active mental engagement with hobbies or activities.

How many times have you thought you were winding down or relaxing when in fact, you were just wasting precious time? Ask yourself, do you actually feel better after procrastinating?

I'm guessing that answer is not - it's just something we do, without really thinking about it.

Procrastination doesn't help us take the action needed for the life you love, it isn't entertaining and it doesn't make us feel good.

Whatever reason you procrastinate, there is little to suggest successful, happy people procrastinate all the time.

It is action, not procrastination, that makes the world go around.

It is also action that will help you achieve the emotional freedom you deserve.

Stop procrastination in its tracks with these EFT phrases … right now!

- I accept I want to procrastinate
- I know procrastination is unproductive
- I can let go of this feeling to procrastinate
- I am in control of my own time
- I know what I need to do

The Seven Ways

We've looked at seven different ways to use tapping to help manage and control your emotions.

These different emotions included anger, impatience, worry, low self-esteem, restlessness, fear of success or failure and procrastination.

To get the most benefit from this book, go back through and underline or highlight those sections which you feel will be most helpful to you.

That way you'll have them ready, for the next time you start to feel your emotions slipping away from you.

SEVEN
CONCLUSION

You've probably heard of the idea of de-cluttering.

De-cluttering is about removing mess and clutter, and bringing order to what was previously disorder.

We all know people who live with clutter in their lives.

Of course, holding onto things isn't necessarily a negative thing.

Holding onto items can bring us comfort.

However, when too much stuff weighs us down, instead of bringing comfort, it can cause anger or distress.

Clutter is not only found in physical items but in our emotions.

Emotions build up and, when we fail to deal with them, cause blockages and hindrances in our lives.

By using EFT and tapping, you can experience breakthrough in your emotions.

By continuing to tap regularly, you can feel a shift or change in your mindset. It may even come in a way you didn't expect.

As long as it results in the feeling of being free, a weight being lifted, and being able to make changes for the positive, you'll know you have made progress!

It may take a while for tapping to become a habit, but once it does, you'll be starting to deal with your emotions, before they build up and cause emotional clutter.

Why not make tapping a new habit for you to use, in every area in your life?

By using it consistently, you'll be giving a wonderful gift to give yourself and those around you.

Happy tapping!

AFTERWORD

If you've found this book useful, please consider leaving a rating or review.

You may also appreciate other books by this author.

CBT for Anxiety : The Psychology of Retraining Your Brain in 21 days

Our thoughts, emotions and behaviours are all connected.

Cognitive Behavioral Therapy offers proven strategies and

techniques for anyone suffers with anxiety, panic attacks or

compulsive disorders to break free by rewiring your brain.

In this book you'll learn how to:

- identify unhelpful thought patterns and negative thoughts
- retrain your brain to help overcome stress and anxiety
- break bad habits that are holding you back from living the life you want
- become calmer and more confident
- break free and feel 100% happier

Regain control over your life with these proven CBT techniques that you

can start using today.

Mindfulness and Meditation for Anxiety - discover proven techniques for helping you deal with your stress and anxiety!

Mindfulness and meditation are not just some hippy idea. They're mainstream, with some of the biggest company names are investing their resources in mindfulness and meditation for their staff.

Studies have shown that mindfulness and meditation can:

- improve the quality and length of sleep
- help focus the mind by reducing distractions
- help you control repetitive thoughts
- improve your memory and mood
- significantly reduce anxiety

By learning how to develop mindfulness and by discovering the power of meditation, you could begin to see the benefits in your life, within weeks.